Anti-Aging Remedies

25 Homemade Essential Oils Recipes

Table of Contents

Introduction

I would like to thank and congratulate you on downloading *"Anti-Aging Essential Oils: Homemade Essential Oil Anti-Aging Remedies!"* You have made a positive choice in downloading this book, it shows that you want to make some changes towards improving the health of your skin by using healthy homemade remedies to do so. More and more people are looking for more natural solutions to helping them remedy many things in life such as skincare treatments that are not filled with chemicals and additives.

It is a smart choice to decide that you are going to start caring for your skin to help it to be as healthy and young looking as it can be. Using natural remedies and treatments that are essential oil based will certainly hep you towards reaching your goal of healthy, wrinkle-free skin. In order to have healthy skin you do not have to spend a small fortune on fancy commercial skin products, many of which have all kinds of ingredients in them that are not natural but synthetic. Now by making the choice to make your own homemade anti-aging skin care products you are not only making a healthy choice for your skin but you will certainly cut down on costs. You will no longer rely on expensive artificial products to treat your skincare needs, instead feel good in knowing you are using homemade products that offer wonderful health benefits to you and your skin!

Chapter 1. You and Your Skin

You and your skin are attached, for life. It goes through different stages such as growth, hormonal changes, puberty right along with you. It is also a great protector, shielding you from infection and illnesses. Your skin is basically the first line of defense that your body has. Your body reveals to the outside world, showing what you have been through, your struggles and stresses in life, and the effects the environment is having on your overall health and well-being. Your body is subjected to the outside environment every time you step out of your front door and into the world that lies beyond it.

As a child you do not think too much of the care of your skin. You enjoy life as a child by doing things such as playing hide-and-seek, riding your bike and other fun activities that you enjoyed as a child. Then you come to the stage in life known as "puberty" this is when you might look in the mirror one day and see your first pimple. You might start to take more notice of your skin, such as you may notice that it seems really dry.

When you get to the stage in life where you "leave the nest' so to speak and begin to support yourself by working you subject your body to the stresses that come with supporting yourself in the world. With the stresses of everyday life your skin also reacts to these stresses. It may begin to feel dry and stretched, it begins to develop wrinkles. You may even notice that you have dark circles under your eyes. This is another phase of the life process that shows the world that you are not getting enough sleep and are stressed.

When you reach your fifties you may begin to notice that your skin is sagging in areas. This occurs due to as your skin ages it loses more and more of its elasticity, this is the trait that allows your skin to bounce back and stay firm and wrinkle-free. Places this is often a problem are areas such as under the chin, skin sags. You begin to start looking and feeling your age. You begin to wonder if there is anyway that you can stop this process or at least slow it down somehow.

What you didn't realize...

Is that you can indeed keep it from occurring by keeping it moisturized, cleansed and toned. One of the first ways to begin this process is to make some healthy changes in your diet. Your skin health starts from within. What you are eating and what those foods contain is going to indeed have an affect on your skin and how it ages.

Processed and fast food...

Most of us living in this fast paced world love convenience. We all to grab a quick bite to eat and rush off to work or attend any other projects on our "to do lists". Often when we are out running around doing errands, rushing here and there, we will stop and grab a quick meal at a fast food restaurant.

 We might come home from a long hard day at work and not feel like preparing dinner, so instead we take out a frozen dinner that is quick and easy to prepare. The big problem with most convenient foods is the chemicals that go into them to preserve them, these end up inside our bodies. Artificial additives can cause your digestive system to rebel, when this occurs this can show in such forms as cold sores, oily skin, bad pimple breakouts. These can all be linked back to the type of food your are consuming in your daily diet.

You can start making better choices in foods by first reading the labels to see exactly what they contain, cutting out greasy foods, junk foods and fast foods. Trade in the burgers and fries for chicken and salad or make a smoothie. Smoothies can be a great way to have a quick healthy meal especially on those days when you are tight for time. They can help to contribute to keeping your skin healthy. They can even begin to reverse some of the skin problems you are dealing with.

Now with a bit of an idea on how to take care of your skin from the inside now you are ready to learn how to care for your skin on the outside.

Chapter 2. Aromatherapy

I am sure you are probably thinking 'what does aromatherapy have to do with my skin?' Well you might think that aromatherapy just covers diffusers and incense, but it also covers things such as facial masks, massage lotions, skin lotions, astringents, cleansers, moisturizers and baths.

Aromatherapy is the aspect of natural health that shows that when it comes to healing it can come through inhaling aromas. The aromas that are made are created by blending essential oils. Essential oils are basically the essence of the plant and often are the most potent of preparations in the holistic field. It takes large quantities of a plant either by a distilling process or pressing the plants for their pure oil. It is this precious oil that is used in several remedies and applications.

The Applications

There is several ways in which one can apply or use essential oils.

1. *Facial Oils*

Facial oils are often used after you have completed the cleaning process of your face to help moisturize it. Depending upon which carrier oil you use and the essential oil blend, they can make both day-time or night-time blends for treating your facial skin.

2. *Soaps*

You can make your own homemade soaps that you can infuse with essential oils for a healthier soap that can cleanse your entire body as well as your face. When you prepare 'melt and pore' soaps at home they will contain more glycerin in them compared to those that you purchase at the store. Glycerin is a natural chemical in the soap that will provide moisture. Many chemically made soaps will actually dry out your skin, due to the fact that many of them do not have glycerin in them.

3. *Astringents*

You can make astringents with witch hazel, a natural cleanser. Depending upon the essential oils that you mix with the witch hazel you will not only cleanse your skin, but you can also rebalance your the pH of your skin. Doing this can in turn reduce oily patches and help to restore the elasticity in your skin.

4. Facial Masks

Often used in spa treatments, facial masks that are infused with essential oils can heal dry, rough skin, treat acne, and help to reduce fine lines and wrinkles. It is usually made by mixing powdered herbs, clay, and other ingredients and then introducing the essential oils of your choice to them.

5. Massage Oil/Lotion

This type of preparation is often used when you are trying to loosen tight muscles, and moisturize skin, and delivering the healing effects of the essential oils at the same time.

6. Bath/Mineral Salts

You can mix your essential oils of choice with Epsom salts and a couple of other minerals and then add this mix into your bath offering you a lovely relaxing therapeutic bath.

7. Diffuser, candle, candle warmer

This application of using essential oils is when you place the 'neat' or undiluted essential oils into a diffuser or candle warmer or the like and warm it to gently release the therapeutic fragrance of the essential oils into the air.

Word of Caution:

Not all essential oils will agree with every skin type. The best way to choose an essential oil that is best suited to you and your needs is to test it on a small patch of your skin. Leave it on there for a few hours and look to see if your skin has reacted to it. If your skin shows that it was not irritated or had an allergic reaction to that particular essential oil then you can feel good in knowing that it will be good choice for you to use in your skin treatments.

Do not use essential oils unless they are diluted, they are very potent and could cause a bad skin reaction if they are not diluted before use. Always use carrier oils to dilute your essential oils.

Chapter 3. Essential and Carrier Oils

In this chapter we will look at some of the most common carrier and essential oils for home remedies and in making beauty products at home. There are a certain set of essential oils that are used most often in beauty and skin care products. I will include the latin name of each essential oil as well so you will know exactly the one that you need.

Common Essential Oils Used in Skin Treatments:

Frankincense Essential Oil

Boswellia carteri

Frankincense essential oil is dated back in history to biblical times, it is often used in incense. However, Frankincense is also used in beauty products to help with blemishes, older skin, dry complexions, and helps in reducing wrinkles

Carrot Seed Essential Oil

Daucus carota

When you read "carrot" you are no doubt picturing the vegetable, and you would be partially correct. It is Wild Carrot. It is also known as 'Queen Anne's Lace'. This essential oil is used in helping to treat wrinkles, and helping to return elasticity and healthy glow to mature skin types.

Lavender Essential Oil

Lavendula angustifolia

Lavender is one of the more widely known essential oils, it is very versatile. You can choose to blend it with most other essential oils. It is good to use in treating acne, age spots, rosacea, and for helping to maintain all skin types by helping to balance pH balance in skin.

Neroli

Citrus aurantium var. Amara

This is also known as 'Orange Blossom', it is known for its ability to tone mature and sensitive skin. It can help to tone the complexion and reduce wrinkles.

Myrrh

Commiphora myrrha

This is another essential oil that has been around since biblical times. Myrrh is often used in aromatherapy for chapped and dry skin, and helps with the maintenance of mature skin, keeping the health and elasticity of the skin.

Orange

Citrus sinesis

Sweet Orange is an essential oil that is often used to bring back the healthy glow to dull skin and will help to balance an oily complexion.

Rose

Rosa x damascena

The Damask Rose is prized for its properties regarding skin and the nervous system. It can help to repair broken capillaries, dry skin, and mature and sensitive complexions.

Patchouli

Pogostemon cablin

This essential oil was added to blends to help with shrinking pores and helping to balance oily skin, and reduce wrinkles.

Sandalwood

Santalum album

This essential oil helps to treat greasy skin, chapped skin and also helps to moisturize skin

Common Carrier Oils Used for Beauty and Skin Care Purposes:

Sweet Almond Oil

This is one of the most popular choices of carrier oils in skin care products. It will help to relieve itching and dryness of your skin. This is a carrier oil that is good for all skin types.

Wheatgerm Oil

This particular oil will help to tone prematurely aged skin and is also good for all skin types. It also diluted in a blend.

Evening Primrose Oil

Primrose is often used to help balance hormones, it is also used to prevent prematurely aging skin. It is often diluted with other carrier oils.

Carrot Oil

Carrot oil is often used for dry skin, prematurely aging skin, and it also helps to rejuvenate the skin. It is diluted with other carrier oils.

Other things you can use

Other ingredients you may use to dilute your essential oils.

Witch Hazel

I touched on witch hazel earlier in the book. You can dilute your essential oils in witch hazel to use as an astringent and other skin tonics.

Bentonite Clay

This mineral clay is used often as a base for facial masks. It is great at helping to detoxify the skin.

French Clay

This type of clay is basically used in the same way as Bentonite clay.

Base Lotion

You can purchase unscented lotions online that you can use to make your own lotions. This is a great way to make moisturizers for your face and body using the essential oils of your choice that you can add to these lotions.

Base Liquid Soap

You can find plain liquid soap online to use to make your own facial cleanser adding essential oils tailored to your skin complexion.

Tips on making your own blends.

I will include recipes in another chapter, but if you are interested in making your own blends and products, here are a few tips.

For every one tablespoon of carrier oil or carrier oil blend add six drops of essential oil. This also will work when you are adding essential oils to soaps and lotions.

Heavier essential oils will be added in smaller amounts than the lighter ones. Heavier essential oils include essential oils that come from herbs and tree saps. Heavier oils are also essential oils that come from tree bark.

The lighter essential oils come from leaves, fruit, rinds and petals. You should add carrier oils in ratios of 10 percent, other than Sweet Almond oil and Apricot oil.

It is best to store your essential oil blends in a dark glass jar. The more light you expose to your essential oils the faster they will lose their effectiveness. Store them in a cool dark place.

Chapter 4. Essential Oils and Aging Skin

As we age, so does our skin. In order to keep your skin healthy as it ages you need to offer it changes in order to keep it healthy, glowing and firm.   In this chapter we will take a closer look at the essential oils that are the most effective in helping with aging skin.

Twenties

To maintain your youthful skin at this age you can use the following essential oils:

- Carrot seed
- Sweet Almond
- Neroli
- Lavender
- Geranium
- Apricot
- Evening Primrose Oil

Thirties

Your body at this age is hitting its peak. Your skin at this point is beginning to show some signs of aging, but you can use the following oils to turn back time:

- Palma Rosa (this oil is used to reduce wrinkles and soften skin)
- Carrot Seed
- Patchouli
- Rose
- Apricot Kernel

- Sweet Almond

- Borage Seed

Forties

At this stage in life you are more mature and so is your skin. You may at this stage notice wrinkles and some dryness to your skin. You may also notice sagging. The following oils can help make improvements to your skins appearance:

- Lavender

- Myrrh

- Carrot Seed

- Neroli

- Rose

- Frankincense

You can use carrier oils such as Wheatgerm oil, Evening Primrose oil and Carrot oil.

Fifties

You will notice more wrinkles appearing, and more sagging, you may even notice age spots. The following oils can help in improving the appearance and health of your skin:

- Neroli

- Lavender

- Carrot Seed

- Myrrh

Using carrier oils such as Borage seed, and Evening Primrose oils work well for this age range of skin.

Chapter 5. Essential Oil Based Facial Cleansers

You have had a long hard day at work and now you are getting ready to cleanse your skin before heading off to bed.

Soaps

Your face is the most sensitive skin compared to the rest of your body, so it deserves special treatment when caring for it. The soaps that you may choose to use on your body may take a real toll on your face.

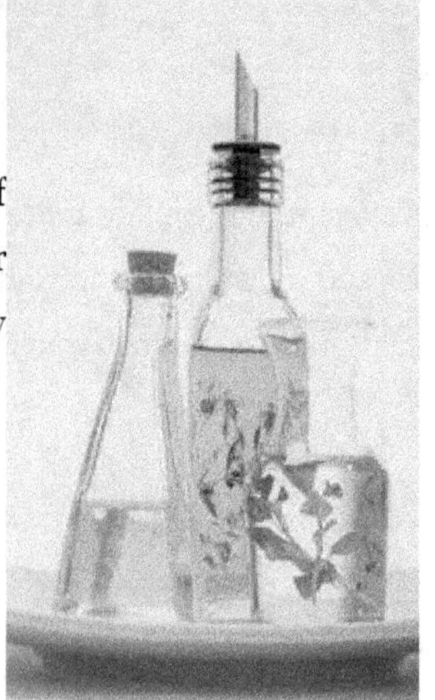

1. Oily Skin Melt and Pour Soap
Ingredients:

- 2 tablespoons of used coffee grinds

- 4 ounces of Goat's Milk Melt and Pour Soap

- 2 tablespoons of oats, ground

- 25 drops of Orange essential oil

- 10 drops of Frankincense essential oil

- 20 drops of Patchouli essential oil

- 20 drops of Geranium essential oil

Directions:

In a double broiler melt your soap. Add in the coffee grounds along with the oats. Pour the soap into molds. Mix the essential oils together then add them into the soap. The coffee grinds will act like an astringent and an exfoliant. The oats will help to absorb any excess oil.

2. *Invigorating Soap*

Ingredients:

- 4 ounces of liquid base soap

- 20 drops of Sandalwood essential oil

- 20 drops of Neroli essential oil

- 30 drops of Orange essential oil

- 30 drops of Peppermint essential oil

Directions:

Add your essential oils to liquid soap in mixing bowl and blend well. Add into soap dispenser after mixing.

3. *Oily Skin Soap*

Ingredients:

- 4 ounces of liquid soap base

- 25 drops of Geranium essential oil

- 25 drops of Carrot Seed essential oil

- 25 drops of Sandalwood essential oil

- 25 drops of Orange essential oil

Directions:

Add your essential oils to liquid soap in mixing bowl and blend well. Add into soap dispenser after mixing.

4. Dry Skin Soap
Ingredients:

- 4 ounces of liquid soap base

- 25 drops of Neroli essential oil

- 25 drops of Rose essential oil

- 30 drops of Lavender essential oil

- 20 drops of Myrrh essential oil

Directions:

Add your essential oils to liquid soap in mixing bowl and blend well. Add into soap dispenser after mixing.

5. Detox Soap
Ingredients:

- 4 ounces of liquid soap base

- 30 drops of rose essential oil

- 25 drops of lavender essential oil

- 30 drops of peppermint essential oil

- 15 drops of Sandalwood essential oil

Directions:

Add your essential oils to liquid soap in mixing bowl and blend well. Add into soap dispenser after mixing.

6. *Soothing Skin Soap*
Ingredients:

- 4 ounces of liquid soap base

- 15 drops of Orange essential oil

- 15 drops of Neroli essential oil

- 10 drops of Myrrh essential oil

- 15 drops of Patchouli essential oil

- 20 drops of Geranium essential oil

- 25 drops of Lavender essential oil

Directions:

Add your essential oils to liquid soap in mixing bowl and blend well. Add into soap dispenser after mixing.

7. *Skin Balancing Melt and Pour Soap*
Ingredients:

- 2 ounces of Goat's Milk Melt and Pour

- 20 drops of Patchouli essential oil

- 25 drops of Geranium essential oil

- 25 drops of Orange essential oil

- 1 tablespoon of Kelp

- 2 tablespoons of coffee grinds

- 2 ounces of olive oil melt and pour

- 20 drops of rose essential oil

- 10 drops of Myrrh essential oil

Directions:

Melt the soap in double broiler. Add in the grinds and kelp, pour soap in molds. Blend essential oils together then add to soap while it is still warm and viable.

8. Melt and Pour Soap for Dry Skin
Ingredients:

- 4 ounces of Olive oil

- 10 drops of Frankincense essential oil

- 20 drops of Myrrh essential oil

- 20 drops of rose essential oil

- 25 drops of Geranium essential oil

- 25 drops of Lavender essential oil

- 2 tablespoons of kelp (natural silicon and minerals that are good for the skin)

Directions:

Melt soap in double broiler, adding kelp pour it into soap molds. Mix and blend your essential oils, add them into the soap while it is still warm and viable.

9. Astringent Base
Ingredients:

- 1 ounce of Apple cider vinegar

- 3 ounces of witch hazel

- essential oils of your choice

Directions:

Use your astringent after you have finished washing with soap as it can remove dirt and oils that the soap may have missed. Once you have mixed your astringent you can add it to a bottle. Use a cotton ball to apply it to your face. Add your essential oils to the apple cider before you add in the witch hazel. The apple cider vinegar will emolliate the essential oils so they will blend or mix better with the witch hazel.

Treatments for the Various Ages

10. Twenties:
Ingredients:

- 1 ounce of apple cider vinegar

- 3 ounces of witch hazel

- 20 drops of Geranium essential oil

- 20 drops of carrot seed essential oil

- 20 drops of lavender essential oil

- 20 drops of peppermint essential oil

Directions:

Mix your essential oils in the apple cider vinegar. Add the infused vinegar to the witch hazel. Place mixture in a dark colored glass bottle. Apply a small amount of astringent using a cotton ball and cleanse your face.

11. Thirties
Ingredients:

- 2 ounces of witch hazel

- 1 ounce of apple cider vinegar

- 1 ounce of rose water (soothes and tones skin)

- 20 drops of peppermint essential oil

- 10 drops of Sandalwood essential oil

- 10 drops of Patchouli essential oil

- 20 drops of rose essential oil

- 20 drops of Palma Rosa essential oil

Directions:

Mix the essential oils in with the apple cider vinegar. Mix the rose water and witch hazel. Mix all of the ingredients together and pour them into a dark glass bottle to store. Place a few drops of mixture on a cotton ball and apply to face.

12. Forties
Ingredients:

- 1 ounce of witch hazel

- 2 ounces of rose water

- 1 ounce of apple cider vinegar

- 20 drops of carrot essential oil

- 10 drops of Frankincense essential oil

- 10 drops of Patchouli essential oil

- 20 drops of lavender essential oil

- 20 drops of Neroli essential oil

Directions:

Mix the essential oils with the apple cider vinegar. Mix the witch hazel and rose water. Add all ingredients into dark glass bottle. Place a few drops of mix on cotton ball and apply to face.

13. Fifties
Ingredients:

- 10 Drops of Geranium essential oil

- 10 drops of Myrrh essential oil

- 10 drops of Sandalwood essential oil

- 20 drops of Neroli essential oil

- 20 drops of lavender essential oil

- 1 ounce of apple cider vinegar

- 1 ounce of witch hazel

- 2 ounces of rose water

- 10 drops of rose essential oil

Directions:

Mix the essential oils with the apple cider vinegar. Mix the witch hazel and rose water. Add all ingredients into dark glass bottle. Place a few drops of mix on cotton ball and apply to face.

Chapter 6. Essential Oil Based Moisturizers

After you have washed, and applied an astringent to your face you may feel that your skin is a bit dry. The next step in your regimen should be to moisturize your skin. This is even more vital if you have oil skin as well as dry. After you have washed your skin it is going to be dry because you have cleansed the dirt and with it your natural oils that help to keep your skin smooth and healthy.

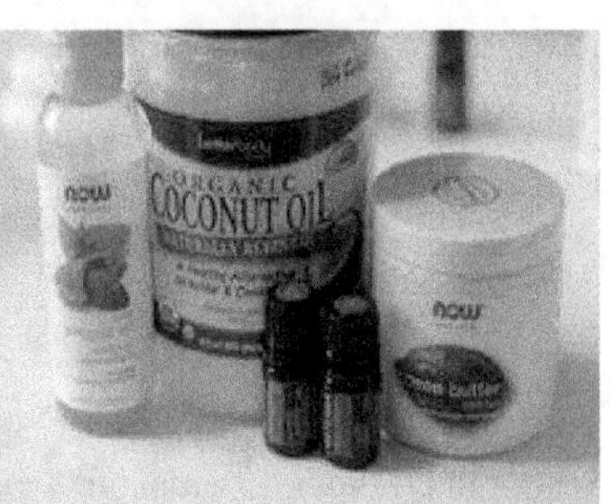

If you have oily skin you may notice that your skin seems to get oily rather quickly after you have washed it. This is due to the fact that your skin is trying to pull moisture back into your skin. There is two ways that you can add moisture back into your skin:

- making a massage oil

- making your lotion

When it comes to some oils they can be lighter than the lotions for your face. These would be a good choice for oily skin types.

Facial Moisturizing oils

14. Twenties
Ingredients:

- 3 1/2 ounces of Apricot Kernel or Sweet Almond oil

- 1/2 ounce of Primrose oil

- 20 drops of Geranium essential oil

- 20 drops of Lavender essential oil

- 10 drops of Sandalwood essential oil

- 10 drops of Orange essential oil

- 10 drops of Carrot seed oil

- 10 drops of Neroli essential oil

Directions:

Mix all of the ingredients together and pour them into a dark colored, glass bottle for storage. Apply to your face using a cotton ball.

15. Thirties
Ingredients:

- 3 1/2 ounces of Apricot kernel oil or Sweet Almond oil

- 10 drops of Carrot Seed essential oil

- 10 drops of patchouli essential oil

- 10 drops of lavender essential oil

- 10 drops of Myrrh essential oil

- 20 drops of Palma Rosa essential oil

- 20 drops of rose essential oil

- 1/2 ounce of Borage seed oil

Directions:

Mix all of the ingredients together and pour them into a dark colored, glass bottle for storage. Apply to your face using a cotton ball.

16. Forties
Ingredients:

- 2 tablespoons of Borage seed oil

- 2 tablespoons of carrot oil

- 10 drops of Frankincense essential oil

- 10 drops of carrot seed essential oil

- 20 drops of Neroli essential oil

- 20 drops of lavender essential oil

- 10 drops of Geranium essential oil

- 10 drops of Orange essential oil

Directions:

Mix all of the ingredients together and pour them into a dark colored, glass bottle for storage. Apply to your face using a cotton ball.

17. *Fifties*
Ingredients:

- 2 tablespoons of Wheatgerm oil

- 2 tablespoons of Evening Primrose oil

- 2 tablespoons of Borage Seed oil, or Sweet Almond or Apricot Kernel oil

- 10 drops of Geranium essential oil

- 10 drops of Sandalwood essential oil

- 10 drops of Myrrh essential oil

- 10 drops of Neroli essential oil

- 20 drops of rose essential oil

- 20 drops of lavender essential oil

Directions:

Mix all of the ingredients together and pour them into a dark colored, glass bottle for storage. Apply to your face using a cotton ball.

Chapter 7. Essential Oil Based Anti-Aging Facial Masks

Using facial masks as a form of treatment for our facial skin will help to detoxify, and tone our skin and help to promote the healing of skin that has been ravaged by the environment and everyday stresses.

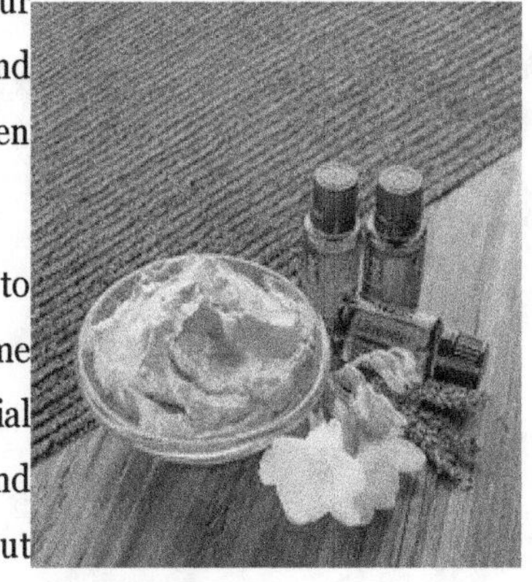

In order to use the masks all you need to do is to moisten three tablespoons of the mask with some warm water and knead into it 6-10 drops of essential oils. Spread the mask evenly across your face and allow it to dry. This should take approximately about 10 minutes. You then re-moisten it to either rinse it off, or you can use it as a scrub before you rinse it off. Always follow a mask treatment with an astringent and then a moisturizer.

Below I have listed the different types of masks that you can use, you can use the essential oil blends from the previous chapter to apply to masks before you apply them to your face.

18. Oily Skin Blend
Ingredients:

- 2 tablespoons of Sweet Almond oil

- 2 drops of Sandalwood essential oil

- 2 drops of patchouli essential oil

- 4 drops of lavender essential oil

- 4 drops of Orange essential oil

Directions:

Add your oil blend to your mask and blend well before applying mask to your face.

19. Dry Skin Blend
Ingredients:

- 1/4 teaspoon of carrot oil

- 2 tablespoons of Apricot Kernel or Sweet Almond oil

- 2 drops of Rose essential oil

- 4 drops of Myrrh essential oil

- 6 drops of lavender essential oil

Directions:

Mix all of the ingredients together and pour them into a dark colored, glass bottle for storage. Apply to your face using a cotton ball.

20. Detox Blend
Ingredients:

- 1 tablespoon of coconut oil, melted

- 1 teaspoon of Borage seed oil

- 2 drops of lavender essential oil

- 2 drops of Orange essential oil

- 4 drops of peppermint essential oil

Directions:

Mix all of the ingredients together and pour them into a dark colored, glass bottle for storage. Apply to your face using a cotton ball.

Here are some mask bases that you can add the above oil blends to.

21. Dry Skin Mask
Ingredients:

1/4 cup of Bentonite clay powder

1/8 of a cup of lavender flowers

1/8 of a cup of Geranium flowers, ground

1/8 of a cup of kelp, powder

22. Oily Skin Mask
Ingredients:

- 1/8 of a cup of Bentonite clay powder

- 1/4 cup of oats, ground

- 1/8 cup of lemon zest, dried

- 1/8 of a cup of kelp, powder

23. Skin Balancing Mask
Ingredients:

- 1/8 cup of Bentonite clay powder

- 1/8 cup of peppermint leaves

- 1/8 cup of orange zest, dried

- 1/8 cup of lavender flowers

- 1/8 cup of French clay powder

24. Detoxifying Mask
Ingredients:

- 1/8 cup of Spirulina

- 1/8 cup of oats, ground

- 1/8 cup of lavender flowers

- 1/4 cup of Bentonite clay powder

Conclusion

I hope that you and your loved ones will enjoy using my collection of anti-aging homemade skin care treatments as much as I do. You can certainly feel good in knowing that these treatments do not contain any harmful chemicals in them, they will help to bring your skin back to a healthy state once again. You will have that healthy glow in no time, once you begin to take care of your skin using these essential oil based skin treatments. There is no better way to care for your skin on the outside than using natural skin care treatments that will not harm your skin but instead help to heal it from the damages it receives being exposed to the harsh elements. Not only will you treating your skin in a healthy manner, but you will also save a ton of money when you stop buying expensive synthetic skincare products. So do your skin and your pocket book a favor and start using these easy to follow anti-aging skincare treatments today!

I want to thank you again for downloading my book, your support of my work means a great deal to me. I hope that I can read a review by you of my book on Amazon! Take care and know you have made a good choice in choosing to try some natural anti-aging homemade skincare recipes.

FREE Bonus Reminder

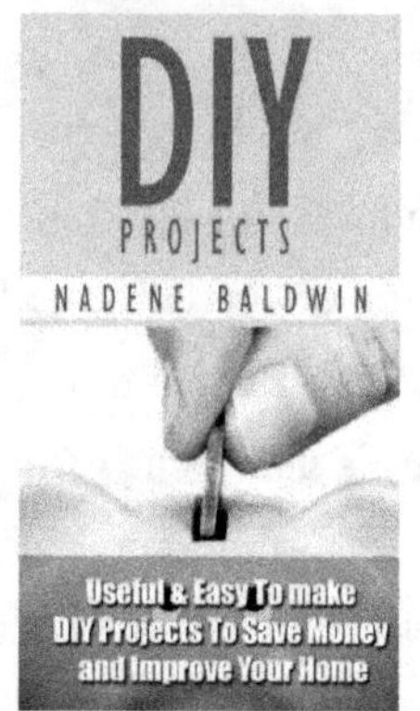

If you have not grabbed it yet, please go ahead and download your special bonus report *"DIY Projects. 13 Useful & Easy To Make DIY Projects To Save Money & Improve Your Home!"*
Simply Click the Button Below

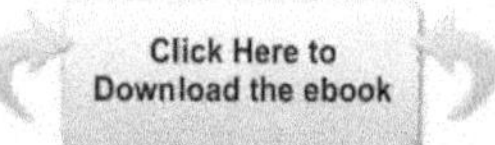

OR **Go to This Page**
http://diyhomecraft.com/free

BONUS #2: More Free & Discounted Books or Products
Do you want to receive more Free/Discounted Books or Products?
We have a mailing list where we send out our new Books or Products when they go free or with a discount on Amazon. Click on the link below to sign up for Free & Discount Book & Product Promotions.
=> Sign Up for Free & Discount Book & Product Promotions <=

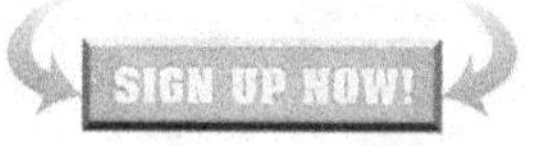

OR Go to this URL
http://zbit.ly/1WBb1Ek

www.ingramcontent.com/pod-product-compliance
Lightning Source LLC
Chambersburg PA
CBHW060824260726
48660CB00003B/1085